SHERRY JARRETT

Sugar is Arsenic

The Sweet Poison That Is Killing You

Contents

Introduction

My Personal Experience with Inflammation from Too Much Sugar

I'll never forget the day I realized just how much sugar was affecting my body. The journey to that realization started months before with a dull ache in my right hand that gradually worsened over time. At first, it was just a minor inconvenience— a slight discomfort when I tried to hold a brush or style my hair with a hair dryer. But soon, it escalated to the point where even gripping my toothbrush was unbearable. The pain was so intense that it felt like my hand was on fire, making it impossible to go about my daily routines.

Desperate for answers, I made an appointment with a hand surgeon. After examining my hand, he ordered an X-ray to see what was going o n. As I sat in the office, anxiously waiting for the results. What if it was something serious? When the surgeon finally returned with the X-ray, he pointed out specific areas in my hand and explained that we were looking at arthritis. My heart sank. He went on to describe a surgical procedure that would involve removing a tendon from my wrist to sew into my hand to alleviate the pain. It was a drastic measure, and the thought of such a complex surgery scared me.

Then, almost as an afterthought, the doctor mentioned something that stuck with me. He said,

"I have patients with far worse arthritis than this, but they don't have any pain." His tone was almost puzzled, as if he couldn't quite understand why some people with severe arthritis had no pain while others, like me, were in agony. It was like he was acknowledging a mystery that he couldn't solve. That comment made me start thinking—why was my pain so severe? What was different about my situation?

I started researching pain in the body and spoke with my chiropractic team about it. I learned that the pain was a result of inflammation and learned how sugar can contribute to it. I finally realized that sugar was slowly poisoning me. It was like a light bulb switched on in my mind, illuminating the countless ways sugar had been wreaking havoc on my body. For years, I had struggled with a range of health issues—unexplained fatigue, stubborn weight gain, frequent bouts of irritability, and a constant battle with inflammation that left me in near-constant pain. I didn't understand why I felt so miserable all the time. I ate what I thought was a fairly healthy diet, but there was a hidden enemy in nearly everything I consumed: sugar.

Let me tell you, sugar isn't just about sweets and desserts. It's lurking in many of the foods we eat daily, often disguised under different names or hidden in foods we might never suspect. The more I dug into the research, the more I realized how insidious sugar truly is. It's not just the obvious offenders like candy and soda. Sugar hides in bread, sauces, dressings, and countless "healthy" snacks. Over time, consuming sugar in these amounts leads to a host of problems: obesity, high blood pressure, fatty liver disease, tooth decay, diabetes, and high cholesterol, just to name a few. But perhaps the most devastating effect of all is the chronic inflammation it causes—a silent killer that manifests as pain and fatigue, robbing you of your vitality and joy.

It wasn't until I decided to eliminate sugar from my diet that I truly began to understand its power. As I removed it from my meals, something amazing happened: my energy levels soared, my mood stabilized, and the chronic pain that had plagued me for years began to dissipate. This transformation was life-changing, and it's why I'm so passionate about sharing this message with you.

In this book, we're going to take a deep dive into the world of sugar—what it is, why it's so addictive, and most importantly, how you can break free from its grip. You're not alone in this, and with the right information and a little determination, you can reclaim your health and happiness. Let's start this journey together, so you can see for yourself how eliminating sugar from your life can lead to profound changes. Believe me, if I can do it, so can you.

1

Chapter 1: What is Sugar?

When you hear the word "**sugar**," what comes to mind? Maybe you think of the white, granulated stuff you put in your coffee or the sweetness of a ripe fruit. But sugar is much more than that. It's a simple carbohydrate that, when consumed, is converted into glucose—a form of sugar that our bodies use for energy. In small amounts, glucose is essential; it fuels our muscles, powers our brains, and keeps us going throughout the day. However, the problem arises when we consume too much sugar, and believe me, most of us are eating far more than we should or we realize.

Let's break down what sugar really is and all the places it hides. First, there are natural sugars, which are found in foods like fruits, vegetables, and dairy products. These sugars, such as fructose in fruits and lactose in dairy, come packaged with fiber, vitamins, and minerals that our bodies need. When eaten in their whole, natural form, these foods provide a slow, steady release of energy, making them a healthy option. But here's where things get tricky: not all sugars are created equal. There's another kind of sugar, added sugars, that are used extensively in processed foods. These sugars have been extracted, refined, and added to foods to enhance flavor or extend shelf life. Think of table sugar, high-fructose corn syrup, and the myriad of other names you'll see on ingredient labels: sucrose, glucose, maltose, dextrose, and more. They all boil down to the same thing: simple carbohydrates that quickly convert into glucose in your body.

Processed foods are often loaded with these added sugars, even in items you wouldn't expect. Breads, sauces, salad dressings, and even so called "health foods" like granola bars and yogurt, often contain high levels of hidden sugars. And here's the kicker: these processed sugars don't come with the natural fibers and nutrients that whole foods do, meaning they hit your bloodstream fast, causing a spike in blood sugar levels followed by a rapid drop.

This rollercoaster effect leaves you feeling tired, cranky, and craving even more sugar a vicious cycle that's hard to break.Then there are the foods that don't taste sweet but quickly convert to sugar in the body, like refined grains. White bread, pasta, and rice are stripped of their fiber and nutrients, causing them to behave like sugar in the bloodstream. Your body digests them quickly, turning them into glucose and sending your blood sugar levels soaring.

Understanding what sugar is and recognizing where it hides is the first step toward taking control of your diet. It's not just about cutting out sweets and desserts—though that's a great start. It's about becoming aware of all the ways sugar sneaks into our diets and learning to make choices that prioritize our health and well-being. In the next chapters, we'll dive deeper into the addictive nature of sugar, how to identify if you're hooked, and most importantly, how to break free. Stay with me; this journey is just getting started, and I promise it's worth every step.

2

Chapter 2: What is Inflammation?

Inflammation is a natural and vital response that your body uses to protect itself from harm. Think of it as your body's internal alarm system, springing into action whenever there's an injury or illness. When you sprain your ankle or get a cut, inflammation is the process that helps your body heal. In these cases, inflammation is a good thing—it signals your immune system to send white blood cells to the affected area to fight off infections and start the healing process. You might notice redness, swelling, heat, or pain; these are all signs that your body is doing its job, working hard to repair damage and defend against harmful invaders.

However, inflammation isn't always a helpful process. Sometimes, your body triggers inflammation even when there's no clear injury or infection. This is known as chronic inflammation, and it can be much more harmful than helpful. Unlike the short, targeted response of acute inflammation, chronic inflammation is a slow, persistent state of alert that can last for months or even years. It occurs when your immune system mistakenly attacks healthy tissues, thinking they are threats, or when it stays activated long after the initial injury or illness has been resolved.

Chronic inflammation can be triggered by a variety of factors. These include long-term exposure to irritants like pollution, untreated infections, autoimmune disorders where the body attacks its own cells, and, importantly, poor diet. A diet high in sugar, processed foods, and unhealthy fats can promote ongoing inflammation in the body, leading to a host of health problems. When inflammation is constantly active, it can damage healthy cells, tissues, and organs. Over time, this damage can lead to serious conditions such as heart disease, diabetes, and cancer, as well as pain and fatigue that can significantly affect your quality of life.

Understanding the difference between acute and chronic inflammation is crucial because it helps us see why managing inflammation, especially through diet and lifestyle, is so important. In the next chapter, we'll explore the link between sugar and inflammation and how reducing sugar intake can be a powerful way to calm this harmful, chronic response. Remember, knowledge is power, and the more you understand about how your body works, the better equipped you'll be to make choices that support your health and well-being.

3

Chapter 3: Sugar is Addictive

Have you ever found yourself reaching for that cookie or craving a soda even when you're not hungry? You're not alone. Sugar has an almost magnetic pull, and it's not just a matter of willpower. It turns out that sugar is actually addictive, much like drugs or alcohol. When you consume sugar, it lights up the reward centers in your brain, releasing a flood of dopamine—a feel-good chemical that gives you a rush of pleasure. This is the same process that occurs with addictive substances, and it's what makes sugar so hard to resist.

Let's dive into how this works. When you eat something sugary, your taste buds send signals to your brain, which in turn releases dopamine in the nucleus accumbens, the part of the brain's limbic system responsible for feelings of pleasure, reward and emotional control. This dopamine release reinforces the behavior, making you want to repeat it. The more sugar you eat, the more your brain craves that dopamine hit, creating a cycle of desire and reward that can be incredibly hard to break. Over time, just like with any addictive substance, you may find that you need more and more sugar to achieve the same pleasurable feeling, leading to increased consumption and dependency.

But sugar addiction isn't just about craving sweets. It comes with a range of symptoms that can affect both your mind and body. If you're addicted to sugar, you might notice that you have strong, uncontrollable cravings for sugary foods, even when you're not physically hungry. You might find yourself eating more sugar than you intended, unable to stop after just one piece of candy or one slice of cake. Often, these cravings can lead to a binge-eating behavior, where you consume large amounts of sugar in a single sitting, followed by feelings of guilt or regret.

Other symptoms of sugar addiction include mood swings, where you feel happy and energetic immediately after eating sugar, but experience a crash soon after, leaving you feeling tired, irritable, and sluggish. You might also notice that you're eating sugar to cope with stress or emotions, using it as a comfort food when you're feeling down or anxious. Physical symptoms can include headaches, fatigue, and a lack of concentration, particularly if you try to cut back on your sugar intake suddenly.

Understanding that sugar is addictive and recognizing the signs of sugar addiction is a crucial step in breaking free from its grip. It's not about depriving yourself or feeling guilty about your cravings; it's about understanding why these cravings occur and finding healthier ways to satisfy your body's needs. In the following chapters, we'll explore strategies for overcoming sugar addiction and reclaiming control over your diet and your health. You don't have to be a slave to sugar, let's find out how to break the cycle and start a new chapter in your journey to wellness.

4

Chapter 4: What Can You Do About It?

Breaking free from a sugar addiction can feel like a daunting task, but the good news is that it's entirely possible with the right approach and mindset. Just like with any habit, overcoming sugar addiction involves understanding your triggers, making intentional choices, and setting yourself up for success. Let's explore some practical steps you can take to reduce your sugar intake and reclaim control over your health.

Step 1: Acknowledge and Understand Your Cravings

The first step in overcoming sugar addiction is to recognize it for what it is—a powerful habit that's been reinforced over time. Acknowledge your cravings without judgment and understand that they're a natural response to the way sugar affects your brain. By identifying the situations or emotions that trigger your sugar cravings, you can start to break the cycle. Keep a food diary for a week, noting what you eat and when you crave sugar. Look for patterns—are you reaching for sweets when you're stressed, bored, or tired? Understanding these triggers is the first step toward changing your habits.

Step 2: Gradually Reduce Your Sugar Intake

Going cold turkey might work for some, but for most people, it's more sustainable to gradually reduce sugar intake. Start by eliminating obvious sources of sugar, like candy, sugary drinks, and desserts. Then, begin to cut back on hidden sugars found in processed foods. Read labels carefully—sugar hides under many names like corn syrup, dextrose, and fructose. Aim to replace these foods with healthier alternatives. Instead of a sugary snack, try a piece of fruit, a handful of nuts, or a yogurt with no added sugars. Your taste buds will gradually adjust, and over time, you'll find that you no longer crave the intense sweetness of sugary foods.

Step 3: Find Healthier Substitutes

One of the keys to kicking your sugar habit is finding satisfying alternatives that won't leave you feeling deprived. Here are a few ideas to get you started: **Fruits and vegetables** are packed with antioxidants, vitamins, and minerals that help reduce inflammation and support overall health. I began to incorporate a variety of colorful fruits and vegetables into my meals, aiming for at least five servings a day. Dark leafy greens like spinach and kale, berries like blueberries and strawberries, and cruciferous vegetables like broccoli and cauliflower became staples in my diet. These foods are rich in antioxidants, which help neutralize free radicals and reduce inflammation.

Choose healthy fats, not all fats are created equal. Healthy fats, such as those found in olive oil, avocados, nuts, and seeds, have anti-inflammatory properties and can help reduce pain and inflammation. I replaced refined vegetable oils with extra virgin olive oil for cooking and salad dressings. I also started adding more omega-3 fatty acids to my diet by eating fatty fish like salmon, mackerel, and sardines. Omega-3s are known for their powerful anti-inflammatory effects and are essential for reducing inflammation in the body.

Refined grains can spike blood sugar levels and contribute to inflammation, so I swapped out white bread, pasta, and rice for whole grains like quinoa, brown rice, and oats. Whole grains have more fiber and nutrients, which help regulate blood sugar levels and reduce inflammation. Including a variety of whole grains in my meals has made a noticeable difference in my energy levels and has helped reduce the inflammation I was experiencing.

Proteins are essential for repair and maintenance in the body, but it's important to choose sources that don't promote inflammation. I began to focus on lean proteins like chicken, turkey, and plant-based sources like beans, lentils, and tofu. These proteins provide the necessary building blocks for the body without contributing to inflammation, unlike red meat and processed meats, which are known to exacerbate it.

Certain herbs and spices have potent anti-inflammatory properties and can be a great addition to an anti-inflammatory diet. I started incorporating more turmeric, ginger, garlic, and cinnamon into my cooking. Turmeric, in particular, contains curcumin, a compound known for its powerful anti-inflammatory effects. Adding these spices to meals not only enhances flavor but also provides added health benefits.

Water is essential for flushing toxins out of the body and maintaining overall health. Staying well-hydrated is important for reducing inflammation and keeping the body functioning optimally. I made it a point to drink plenty of water throughout the day and included herbal teas like green tea and chamomile, which also have anti-inflammatory properties.

Step 4: Getting Started

By making these dietary changes and focusing on whole, nutrient-dense foods, I was able to significantly reduce the inflammation in my body and the pain that came with it. An anti-inflammatory diet is not just a temporary fix but a sustainable way to nourish your body and support long-term health. If you're struggling with inflammation or looking to improve your overall well-being, I encourage you to explore this way of eating. It can make a world of difference. A world without pain caused by sugar.

This is a 7 day eating plan that can help you ease into your new way of eating. This begins with a foundational food that is a vegetable bone broth. It's purpose is to give you an easy concentrated source of nutrition. It is full of minerals, glucosamine, chondroitin and gelatin.(Find the recipe below).

Breakfast (same for 7 days)
8 oz carrot juice
2 hard boiled eggs

1 tablespoon coconut oil

Fresh fruit i.e, papaya or pineapple

BETWEEN MEALS DRINK 2 CUPS OF BONE BROTH

Lunch (same for 7 days)

Protein Drink (whatever protein powder you like) and add Coconut Milk to taste

Salad - chopped salad with 4 of the following vegetables and 1 type of nut (no peanuts)

Artichokes, asparagus, avocado, beans, bean sprouts, beets, broccoli, brussel

sprouts, cabbage, carrots, cauliflower, cucumbers, celery, endive, fennel, fresh

green peas, kale, kohlrabi, onions, parsley, radishes, spinach, turnips.

Salad dressing - ½ c olive, avocado or grapeseed oil, ¼ c organic apple cider vinegar,

¼ c organic lemon juice. Serve 8 level tablespoons with the salad.

1 tablespoon coconut oil

Fresh Fruit of your choice

BETWEEN MEALS DRINK TWO CUPS OF BONE BROTH

Dinner (same for 7 days)

6 oz Fish or chicken (baked, broiled or grilled)

Cooked vegetables, 2 of kind previously listed saute with olive, avocado, grapeseed or

coconut oil

Coconut oil 1 tablespoon

Fresh fruit of choice

If you're still hungry, eat fresh fruits and vegetables and drink the bone broth

Recipe 1: Vegetable Bone Broth

2 16oz (approximately) high quality bone broth

7 carrots cut up fine

1 bunch of celery cut up fine

Small bunch of parsley cut up fine

Bunch of Spinach cut up fine

1 Vidalia Onion cut up fine

2 Tablespoon Apple Cider Vinegar

ADD Salt, pepper, cumin and turmeric to taste

Pour bone broth into a large crock pot, add fresh vegetables and boil until desired

consistency. Store in the refrigerator.

Recipe 2: Earth Milk

You will need a strong blender to ensure you get a smooth, creamy end product.

Fill blender with 5 hefty handfuls of mixed greens (a kale, chard, spinach or power

greens mix is good) and a handful of parsley

Add 2 generous pinches of salt

Add 3-4 tbsp. virgin coconut oil

Shake some cinnamon in (your discretion)

Add drizzle of pure vanilla extract

Add stevia or favorite sweetener to taste

Add 2 scoops of protein powder

Boil a cup of water in a saucepan and add 3 tea bags of your tea and let steep 5 minutes

Remove tea bags and add enough water to the saucepan until the water is no longer

boiling hot, but very warm. Not cold, Not hot, warm!

Add this to your blender and blend for about 2 minutes. Do

not blend too long and heat
up the drink.
Remove from the blender and pour into a 64 oz. container, add pure cold water until
full. Put on a lid and shake well.
Refrigerate and drink freely

Recipe 3: Berry Bliss Smoothie

Ingredients:
1 cup unsweetened almond milk
1/2 cup fresh or frozen berries (strawberries, blueberries, or raspberries)
1/2 banana
1 tablespoon chia seeds
1 handful of spinach (optional)
Instructions:
Combine all ingredients in a blender.
Blend until smooth.
Pour into a glass and enjoy!

Recipe 4: Sweet Potato and Quinoa Salad

Ingredients:
1 large sweet potato, peeled and diced
1 cup quinoa, cooked
1/4 cup chopped walnuts
1/4 cup dried cranberries (no added sugar)
2 cups mixed greens
2 tablespoons olive oil
1 tablespoon balsamic vinegar
Salt and pepper to taste
Instructions:

Preheat oven to 400°F (200°C).

Toss the diced sweet potato with a tablespoon of olive oil, salt, and pepper. Roast for

20-25 minutes until tender.

In a large bowl, combine the cooked quinoa, roasted sweet potato, walnuts,

cranberries, and mixed greens.

Drizzle with the remaining olive oil and balsamic vinegar. Toss to combine.

Serve and enjoy!

Step 5: Build a Support System

Breaking a sugar addiction isn't easy, and it's important to have support. Share your

goals with friends or family members who can encourage you and help hold you

accountable. You might also consider joining a support group or finding a health coach

or nutritionist who can guide you through the process.

Step 6: Be Kind to Yourself

Finally, remember that overcoming sugar addiction is a journey, not a race. There will

be times when you slip up, and that's okay. Don't beat yourself up over a bad day.

Instead, acknowledge it, learn from it, and get back on track. Every step you take

towards reducing your sugar intake is a step towards better health and a happier, more energetic you.

By understanding your cravings, making gradual changes, and finding delicious

alternatives, you can break free from sugar and enjoy a healthier, more balanced life.

Remember, you're not alone in this journey—take it one day at a time, and soon you'll

find that sugar no longer has control over you. Let's take this journey together, and

make a change for a better future!

creating a cycle of cravings and consumption that can be incredibly hard to break. But you've also learned that breaking free from this addiction is possible. With a deeper understanding of how sugar affects your brain and body, you're now equipped with the knowledge and tools you need to make a change. We've gone through practical steps to reduce your sugar intake, find healthier alternatives, and take back control of your diet and your life. You have the power to transform your relationship with food and take control of your health.

Remember, this isn't about perfection. It's about making small, consistent changes that add up to a significant difference in your overall well-being. You have the knowledge, the recipes, and the strategies to make lasting changes. So now it's time to take action! Embrace this straightforward, no-nonsense approach to living a healthier life. You have the ability to change your life forever,one step, one meal, one day at a time.

As you embark on this journey, don't forget to share your experience. Leave a review of this book on Amazon and let others know how this tool has helped you achieve a better life. Your feedback can inspire others to make the same positive changes you're making. Thank you for taking this journey with me. Here's to a healthier, happier you. **Now go out there and make it happen!**

Resources **Australian Healthcare Provider HCF** https://www.hcf.com.au/health-agenda/food-diet/nutrition/impact-of-sugar-on-body

Cleveland Clinic https://my.clevelandclinic.org/health/symptoms/21660-inflammation

ARDU Recovery Center https://www.ardurecoverycenter.com/why-is-sugar-considered-a-drug/#:~:text=Research%20shows%20that%20our%20brains,that%27s%20associated%20with%20emotional%20control.

Google Search https://www.google.com/search?q=what+are+the+symptoms+of+sugar+addiction&oq=what+are+the+zymtoms+of+sugar+addi&gs_lcrp=EgZjaHJvbWUqCQgBEAAYDRiAB DIGCAAQRRg5MgkIARAAGAoYgAQyCAgCEAAYFhgeMgoIAxAA GIYDGIAEGIoFMgoIBBAAGIAEGKIEogEJMjIxNjBqMGooqAIBsA IB&client=ms-android-samsung-rvo1&sourceid=chrome-mobile&ie=UTF-8

Cleveland Clinic https://health.clevelandclinic.org/how-to-sto

p-sugar-cravings

5

Conclusion

Congratulations on reaching the end of this book and taking the first steps toward a healthier, more vibrant life. You've learned about the devastating effects that consuming too much sugar can have on your body, from weight gain and high blood pressure to diabetes and fatty liver disease. Most importantly, you've discovered how sugar fuels inflammation—a silent, chronic condition that can cause pain and damage to your body over time.

We explored how sugar is addictive, creating a cycle of cravings and consumption that can be incredibly hard to break. But you've also learned that breaking free from this addiction is possible. With a deeper understanding of how sugar affects your brain and body, you're now equipped with the knowledge and tools you need to make a change. We've gone through practical steps to reduce your sugar intake, find healthier alternatives, and take back control of your diet and your life. You have the power to transform your relationship with food and take control of your health.

Remember, this isn't about perfection. It's about making small, consistent changes that add up to a significant difference in your overall well-being. You have the knowledge, the recipes, and the strategies to make lasting changes. So now it's time to take action! Embrace this straightforward, no-nonsense approach to living a healthier life. You have the ability to change your life forever—one step, one meal, one day at a time.

As you embark on this journey, don't forget to share your experience. Leave a review of this book on Amazon and let others know how this tool has helped you achieve a better life. Your feedback can inspire others to make the same positive changes you're making. Thank you for taking this journey with me. Here's to a healthier, happier you! **Now go out there and make it happen!**